THE HISS

BY

ALMA BLAIR

Published by Alma Blair aka Kate Dobrowolska
Publishing partner: Paragon Publishing, Rothersthorpe
First published 2023
© Alma Blair aka Kate Dobrowolska 2023

Cover artwork: Lewis Sharpe

ISBN 978-1-78222-979-7

Book design, layout and production management by Into Print
www.intoprint.net
01604 832149

There is a hero within.

"A strong-willed soul"

1.

Younger Years

6 Years Old

"Faster, faster!" Brenna giggles as brother Ty pushes the swing
with one hand while looking at his phone. Her legs buckle backwards,
her stomach squeezes tightly, she throws up a mass of noodles,
chicken, and carrots. *"Sorry!"* she squeals.

Most brothers will moan or shout at their sibling, but he shrugged his
shoulders thinking it was a waste of mum's dinner, Ty is very relieved
the food landed on the grass and not on his sister.

Brenna idolises Ty he is always available for her. She likes watching him
play football at the park. Sometimes it feels like hours waiting for the
game to finish so she makes daisy chains dodging the ball every time it
lands too close. She is a nervous child especially when watching a
friendly football match if the ball strays it could hit her in the face.

The boys use her as a ball girl, but it seems a long way to fetch it.

"HURRY UP!" an echo of ungrateful teenage boys' annoyance
urge her to run after the ball.

The bush leaves ripple with a gusty breeze blow
as Brenna reaches for the ball under the thicket,
walking away hugging the ball, she turns around
and hears a hiss.

"What's that noise?" she runs to Ty to tell him.

Ty reassures her, there are no hissing creatures in the park,
she is imagining things. Football game over, his side has won,
he gives little sis a croggy home. Brenna loves her big brother,
everyone calls him Ty he does not like his name Tynan.

"Why are you late for tea?" Dad is angry over nothing,

Ty huffs, he cannot wait to leave home because dad irritates him.

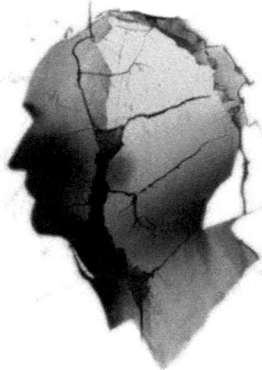

2.

Young Thoughts

8 Years old

Brenna lies in bed at night shadows loom in every corner leaping threats that consume her into panicking, increasing her anxiety and cheeks flushing crimson. Insecurities are rife, her father's mood swings cause her anxious moments.

She cries out for mum most nights her continuous nightmares create heat sweats and nervous shivers. Mum rises sleepily to rescue her dream fears, cuddling her warmly and soothing her head with soft strokes, the smells of powdery talcum cause Brenna to sneeze, mum never wears perfume just soap and talc, perfume is too expensive to buy, and she cannot remember Mum having any gifts given. *Ever!* Mum is so selfless.

Brenna has a hidey den under the table to hide from Dad's unpredictable moods, her brother has a busy social life with his school mates, she feels lonely without his company. The Hiss followed Brenna home after the football game, he clings like a shadow and wants her to be his friend, but she prefers to have a little sister or brother to grow up with. Mum firmly replies *'No!'* when Brenna asks her for a sibling.

Mum lays a picnic dinner on a large tray, with sandwiches, crisps, an apple, banana, and the best tasting chocolate crunchy biscuits. Brenna loves sitting under the table to eat, the blue cotton tablecloth hangs low almost touching the food. She invites the Hiss to join her, but it never appears on request, he only makes a noise when emotions are rife.

Mum carries orange juice in a big plastic jug, Brenna insists on pouring the drink herself. The jug is too heavy to hold upright, and she accidently drops it, the sticky liquid soaking into her clothes, and puddling messy drips everywhere.

Dad is home from a long day at work and he sees the mess!
There will be trouble now!

He is very tired; he travels to work on a motor bike in all weathers, his musty pungent sweaty feet smell rank.

Throwing his shoes and socks off randomly he asks mum to bring him a hot soapy basin to soak his feet clean then sits heavily into his armchair, the one *no one else dares to sit in*, his legs shaking from stress and working long hours.

Brenna feels his tiredness and his negative energy building up, it stirs her emotions up too, they both clash in vibes and character. He unpredictably lurches out of the chair clenching his fists into a tight ball, then sits down again shouting to mum to come and clean the wet floor.

Brenna thought he was coming for her! She really did!

Mum rushes in to rescue the moment carrying a large enamel basin, warm towel, with soapy bubbles to soothe dad's feet so he calms down, then she cleans the floor with a hot wet tea towel, Brenna bubbles tears with a sniff:

"Sorry! Sorry!" she repeatedly whimpers before running upstairs to change her clothes. She wishes dad will show her a bit of love, instead of acting agitated, he never hugs anyone.

In the corner of the room the hissing shadow is angry from behind the sofa, he always emulates everyone's mood issues, and can be scarier to hear than dad. The family do not hear the hiss or see him, so she must be special? Dad is a good man, a hardworking man, but he is constantly nervous and volatile shouting too much daily.

When the shadow stops hissing, he makes spit noises, and bangs a slow thump on the wall, the floor, against a window, and rattling the door. There is always a long dark shadow following the hiss.

The Hiss never shows himself when Brenna calls for him, he ignores her, *why?* She has named the creature 'my sad friend' because he always hides, and if he ever introduces himself to her, she will ask him if he is happy? Everyone needs a friend.

If Hiss feels upset, she is happy to hug him better, but she doesn't know what he looks like. Brenna's family are not very tactile, loving feelings are lost.

Brother Ty left home it has upset Brenna deeply. She misses him, one minute he was there for her, then he disappears without telling her. Just her and mum against dad's dominant unhappy roar.

She feels let down, but Mum said Ty found a job in another area and was living there.

Shouting is not good it really is not. Brenna wants to scream back every time father raises his voice, but stays silent, in fear of him smacking her with his heavy leather belt because a back chat can lead to a mountain avalanche of torrid nastiness. Father does not apologise either, he thinks it is *OK*.

She feels happier at school, which is close to home, and her little black cat 'Misty' follows her down the road to make sure she gets there safely, then Misty goes back home, and waits for her on the garden gate when school closes. Pets are good companions in sadness.

9

Dad does not like Misty at all! he says she pees in his vegetable plants, when most cats pee in a neighbour's garden, but mum insists on having pets for company, to focus on them rather than dad's mood illness. Jesse is part of the family too he is a little terrier dog, and she has trained him to do tricks.

The Hiss still hides in dark corners, but his shadow is becoming much bigger and his energy stronger and a strange smog smell is in the air or is it mum burning food again? because she is very forgetful and depressed frequently.

It is easy to catch father's mood bug. The Hiss spits in the night and makes noises like a kettle over boiling. Brenna wakes up most nights, she constantly feels tired in school with poor sleeping rhythms because of bad tension in the home environment. Her head feels overactive and concentration dreamily scatty. She hopes her imaginary friend will tell her who he is.

One day.

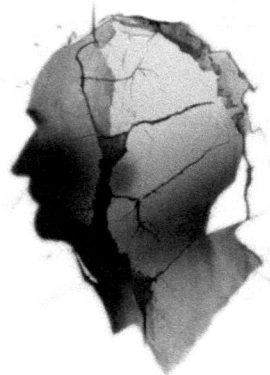

3.

Teenage Sadness

13 years old

All sorts of strange thoughts flutter through Brenna's mind,
She over thinks in abundance her body movements hyperactive with
irritational tetchy mood swings daily. Brenna's fraught relationship
with her father is tense because she throws her anger back at him.
Her aunty died; Brenna feels her slip away in a dream in the early hours.
She feels strong intuitive thoughts deep in her gut, she screams aloud:

"Aunty is dead! She is dead in her bed!"

Aunty died the same time as Brenna awoke.
This is the moment psychosis kicked in badly, full blast with no
turning back.
A tail shadow emerges from the wardrobe slightly ajar, thumping,
swaying, no head, or body, just a strange chomping sound and a
gnawing gnashing of invisible teeth, Brenna is in shock her heart
broken, aunty is not coming back, she wails uncontrollably which
echoes from the wardrobe in sympathy,
in heart pain she grieves:

"It is your fault! Your fault!

11

Show yourself Hiss devil! My Aunty is dead you killed her!"

A hiss eerily whispers back:

"I wasn't there!"

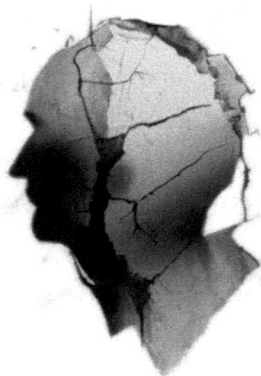

4.

Teenager Anxiety

16 years old
Brenna's Diary Extract
Winter

"Is there a way to let go of the demons that cling to the brain?
Things touch me, silent things, negative vibrations in the air, noises that others
do not hear, strangers talking outside my ear and images unclear.
Voices in the mind, the voices seem true, actions I do not like from other people too.
The environment is alien, each room shows fear, wherever I go a demon is near, now
there is a hiss gate keeper attached to me luring me to his corner silently. He has not
shown his face, but I know he is not human, so he is a creature from hell who has
come to doom me and curse me into
a cess pit full of lying snakes, they will wrap their tails around me,
then choke my throat. The world is one living lie.
There is no reality, only immortality survives.
The flesh is an avatar a cover for sin when flesh rots away
the soul flies away. A good journey? or a bad one?
it depends on what people have done with their life in the past.
I am going to try hard to keep busy in work because higher education
does not suit me and I have a boyfriend to settle down with too,
we have not known each other long and we are both young.

Is this love? Or an escape from my manic dad?
The hiss is more profound, shadows create dark vibrational waves,
and now I hear him move around me with the sound of his tail swishing furiously,
the crunching becomes noisier, and then he **bites!**
He must be very hungry! to want my throat."

Brenna chokes and spits bloodied phlegm out.

Damn the chest infection!

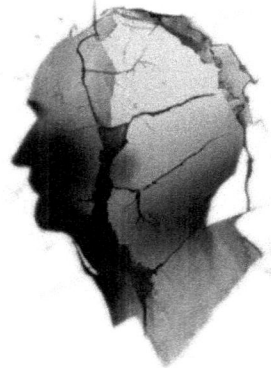

5.

Alienated Life

Adulthood
Diary Extract
Spring

"I marry and the Hiss is my bridesmaid, I am hoping that my imaginary
friend will be fraught with jealousy and abandon our friendship?

No! *he likes being a gooseberry between husband and me!*
Hiss has decided that he will scare the other half and we can have an eternal
triangle of hell between the three of us, and when children
come along, my creature friend will devour their wholesome minds,
bite off their heads and chew them up, eating humans for a living
is nothing new with wildlife, nor is spitting out the remains.
It has not happened yet! My emotions feel hiss now, I feel his weight,
he is a heavy creature, I feel his ugliness, he is not pretty at all.
He makes me shiver and spikes my eyes to bawl. My parents died
when I still needed their support, so now hiss is my guide.
My husband has creature thoughts that warp his mind. I do not think
he has worked out who the gruesome mind creature is. Yet!
He hides inner demons that I never knew he had. Ignorance in not
having self-awareness of your own personality issues is a sad virtue,
this makes hubby more mind abusive towards me, and I feel in despair.

His facetious alter-ego has dismembered my troubled head, I realise that I married in haste. Not even hiss is saving me, he watches me when I am intimate with my man, there is always three of us in the love nest, and an army of demonic viewers peering from within our tormented unhappy conscious state. This marriage will not work, husband is not my type of man!"

I feel trapped in a loveless relationship.

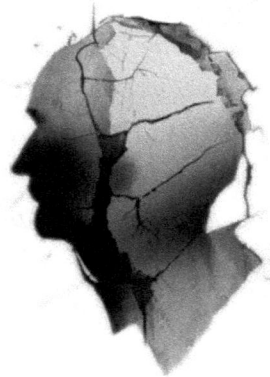

6.

Spat Out

Muddled Adult
Diary Extract
Summer

"I am now in my twenties decade and having no joy within marriage.
Husband wants a family while he is still young, and my inner gut tells me
this will go wrong. The desires in man to produce offspring is strong,
and I feel I must play along. To keep him happy! Sadly!
Hiss is encouraging me to be productive he starts to croak,
I am sure I can hear a voice from his throat.
I know as soon as I feel my growing belly, the child will be a special treat,
not for us as parents but for hiss, who wants human food to eat!
Am I performing an exorcist? or a sacrifice that is odd?
The baby is not even born yet, and I am offering it
to the hissing Gatekeeper God.
My feelings of love for the imminent first birth have yet to come,
no instant bonding with my little son.
The baby is born in a hurry, four hours of pain and he arrives
in orgasmic glory. I look at this tiny creation, and do not
believe he is mine I am worried that if I take him home
the hiss will be jealous and ruin my son's life.

Have I lost all my senses? the environment is surreal,
I feel limp and lifeless floating lightly in the air.
No loving feelings within me, just my eyes proud from afar,
so, why does the Hiss want to pickle my baby in a jar?

Hiss is looking in the baby pod cot, his tongue darts in and out,
the hissing from my keeper turns into slush! He turns around
slurping my belly, my feet are turning into jelly,
his claws digging in, scratching my umbilical hole.

"You cannot have the cord the nurse has taken it
you evil monster!"

I pierce a scream! and hiss turns his attention
to the baby wrapped in a sheet.

"HE WANTS MY BABY!" *I thunderously shout,*
causing medical staff to run towards me in a panic.
They strap me to my bed and take my baby away,
until I can calm the anxiety attack.
My beautiful little son, so small so perfect in every way,
what sort of world has he entered in?
all along hiss is following me slowly like a shadow devil
of flaming sin. I shiver, I shake, I am exhausted, even though
the delivery was quick and neat, then a nurse administers a potion
through my veins to wipe my memory clean. I fall into a deep sleep.
Hiss is still in my nightmares, spitting, cursing, and biting.
Will I wake up? and still have a body? Or will my life stay a permanent
haze? I am drowsy from pills, hiss is gnawing into my brain, he is burying his
tongue in my ears and confusingly I mutter:

18

"Stop!" I am a maniacal prisoner locked within a mind which is turning to rot.
I am a floating ghost my eyes opaquely stare.
Hiss is thirsty he sucks my blood dry, and when I become dehydrated, shrivelled
then drained, he takes me back to his dingy lair, gazing lovingly,
at his trophy with contentment but does he really care?

I awaken my senses thinking; *"I hope we bond well before this happens!"*

Will I ever? ever?
put this shadow monster in a grave to bury his need to dominate,
if I do not, then I will die in defeat! and an explosion of hissing beasts will
rule the Earth. The beast is a leach that grasps my consciousness
to freeze my memory, then he lets go and treats me like a lifelong mate.
What have I done to deserve all of this? All I want is love in this sad world!
I feel brain dead inside. No feeling at all in my body and mind,
I will not reach the dawn theta awakening, because I am
destined for Hiss hell for sure, this time!"

She struggles with crazy thoughts.

"The doctors say to write unbalanced thoughts away
and throw them in the wind. I will try it,
and see if it releases my weird head sins"

7.

Wilderness

Oblivious Mum
Diary Extracts
Autumn

"I gave birth to another child quite quickly,
it is wrong of me to feel insecure.
I need to breed for the beasty long shadow
as he thirsts for a family of four.
I spend time in therapy care, unaware,
it is a place that will keep me safe with locked doors.
I wish this is true, but no! as I hear the clamping of loud jaws,
feeling swing waves of a breeze forward and back?
No pets allowed in here! I panic attack, once more.
My children are so young, they need me,
and keep asking dad, when is mum coming back?
The husband brings them to visit,
his face is tired, annoyed, and drawn.
He does not know his unkempt wife anymore.
The beast might as well devour me whole,
and stamp my bones into the floor.
I become lost so lost in darkness I cannot claw a way out.
the Hiss, now the beast, is silently waiting to catch me,
then he will **spit me out for sure!"**

8.

A Decade Wasted

Tormented
Diary Extract
Spending time in the hospital

"Ten years of institution, ten wasted years.
I am usually ok in summer and winter, then lose my way
in spring and fall. The humongous hiss beast behind my back,
is stalking me once more. The clock changes time twice a year,
it pushes forward then pushes back.
This triggers levers in my brain waves,
jumbling thoughts bonking mad.
I am hardly sleeping, running around, delirious with exploding grandeur,
paranoia is gripping, and while I am sitting, hiss is rocking my chair.
The tiredness, lethargy, forgetfulness adding burdens to my issues,
and when I think of positive things, the dark souls insist that
I undress, and scantily dance naked in the eye of light.
I hook up to manic rhythmic waves while my husband panics inside,
to me in my vision he is looking forlorn with sad zombie eyes.
Off to the slaughter I must go, quietly, meekly, or husband will
be angry and more, and there skulking in the hallway, hiss is
having a convenient piss! vomiting blood on the front door.
Husband feels agitated and holds his head in despair!
His love for me has lost its appeal. My whole life is now surreal,

our lives ruined by this mood infestation, to cap it all we have
tumbled and stalled swimming in mentally melted manifestation.
The gloom of a marriage in demise has made me realise,
that the man I married is not true. I rescue myself when the
mind has blown by listening to music all night through.
The problem is it deafens the ears as I do not hear the sound,
the whole house shakes and the hallow 'weeny' awake,
crying for me to stay and not go away, my young children are loud.
But wait... where is my mate? The one who hisses and spits?
He is thumping the door again, the beastie eyes are gleaming,
he is sizzling and steaming at the thought of a hospital stay.
The same patients return, each cycle each year, and I am
no different too. I can imagine we are all in the same mental motion,
winding Satan's hypnotic tune. The carousel of fire, brimstone, and ash,
will drive us further up the wall, and with all the beasts on patients backs,

I know mine is the king of them all!

Husband drives me to the crazy hotel, the cars on the road salute
my ill health, the traffic lights change sequence in line with my vision,
I creepily smile to myself. I feel like a queen No! a goddess for sure,
I control all the traffic flow, and guess who is nodding in the boot of the car
with his tail thumping slow.? My soul mate will guard me in this
horrendous place, it will be hard to keep him under control.
For every person who shows disgrace, the Hiss will relish them all.
I do not even receive a kiss goodbye as husband gives the suitcase
to the nurse then scurries out of the door. Loveless wimp!
I am sad in my eyes, wiping a tear, while Hiss breaths in my negative despair,
how do I cope with delusions and more? as I really hate who I am.

The nurse on the ward authoritative and cold, registers me in.
I fall asleep with one stab of a jab, and the Hiss curls into a wall.
He will be back to curse when the sun smiles and warmly appears.
I slip into slumber hearing the nurse shout:

"Medication is here!"

I am slowly fading into the sand man's cave, and hoping that
the hissing beast watches my back. I cry in mind pain...

"I hate it here! I want my bed back!"

a creepy tail prods me in my fearful tummy,
I hear a spat and words hiss out"

"I want you! my manic mummy!"

I have lost my senses! Hello crazy world, and 'mind' land of rhyme.

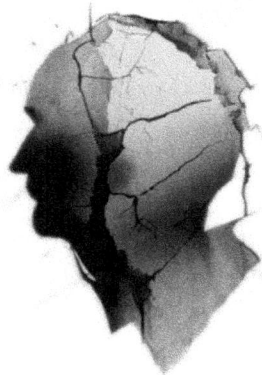

9.

CALAMITY!
Which Season Is It?

Diary Extract
Get me out of here!

"It is hard to get out quickly once locked away.
The days drag by, there is no time, and the patients have little to say.
There is one that drools and another who gabbles,
and three sitting in silence as if dead!
An elderly man asks me politely and kindly:

"Please can I cum inside your bed?"

Why are there mixed wards between the communal room?
It makes me scared to go to sleep in case I have a visitor.
Hiss has started to mind control choosing his prey each day.
One person smashes his way out of a window, the blood spitting
curdling scream makes me shiver. Hiss whispers to me he pleads guilty,
he gently nudged him through the glass 'apparently'!
I look at my hiss guardian in disbelief the window strongly protected
with heavy tubular bars of metal.

"You call that a gentle nudge?
The bars are mangled and bent wide open!"

Hiss awkwardly snuffs, then heavily stomps away to seek his
next hallucinating victim.

A young woman in the kitchen is shouting in delirium,
she is stabbing herself! The knifes are plastic and blunt,
she keeps chiselling her wrists with force 'the silly cunt'.
A young man is crying profusely in the corner, but no one helps,
and a lady named Dot has lost the plot because she is high as a hell!
What is she on? Most pills sedate why can't I have one?
There is a moan from the next room the distraught person must go
to treatment room today. If anyone goes there, they lose their crown
to blasts of electricity wired. At least they do not pay for it!
Hiss beast knows that he will soon have meat, he is waiting for them to fall.
If they give in their 'will' he hunts them out, and they disappear for ever more.
He battles the patient's monsters and always wins, then claims each death as
his own, he brings me the trophy of blood in his teeth, in my nightmare zone.
I am still waiting for the day for him to materialise as a real creature
then my bubble can burst into reality.
I still do not know who the Hiss really is, he must have dual personality?
It is easy to multiply delusions because the mind fragments when ill,
it is like fixing a jigsaw while flying high in a sky, and the pieces fall towards
gravity! Hiss appears with a head in his mouth, and I cannot believe what he
has done, I realise that the man who fell out of the window has found his wings
and now his journey has moved on.
I shout out to the nurse:

"When is it medication time? I need stronger pills!

"In an hour dear, lie down and chill!" the nurse laughs answering back.
"They time keep too well" I think to myself, as I go back to my bed to rest

Hiss secretly muffles a sneer:

"I will join you"

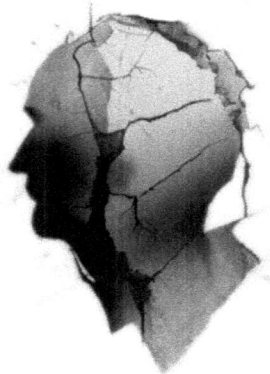

10.

Emotions. Flashback in Time!

Diary extract fantasies

"*As a child from the age of 5yrs to 14yrs old, fantasies in my head were rife, they compensated for an over-active mind and sexual feelings which rocketed sky high. I am sure I was born to scream out:*

"OHHHHHHHHHH!"

Sexual fantasies dominated my life filled with monster fantasy thoughts, the more they are weird the better the euphoric feelings flow.
I never watch horror movies I do not like mind disturbing suspense or thrills involving hurting and mutilating, however characters of monsters I relish in sexual explosive finger action; Frankenstein, Godzilla, King Kong, Dracula, anything out of character and deformed, stimulate my senses, but then the aggression seeps in, one cannot be an ever ready sexually ripe plum, without taking a breath and becoming nasty! Bipolar one recognised at the age of twenty-one and my future hopes of a smooth ride through living, turned into a raunchy ride of hell. Why does the medical profession talk in terms of Euphoria when one is high or manic? As if it is a state of oblivious emotion? when really the culprit is plainly sexual need gone wrong! I can only imagine that to tell people that they are overly sexually active in thought, creates a sad ambience of being a freak and make oneself feel self-conscious, sexual feelings are so personal to an individual but not everyone is a sexual predator! There are other forms of Bipolar, all humans are individuals.

Hiss listens intently to my conscience self-talk, because verbally I am just gabbling like a goose, or a gobbling turkey! I have noticed he is lying at my feet under the covers, chewing the fungus off my hereditary toe-nail disease. But hey! I am ecstatic! as I can see his face forming at last! He does not look as scary as I thought. The rest of him is a mist except for the end of his tail. I do feel a little excited that I am growing a monster companion, who will protect me. The beast finishes his Alpha-Keratin meal, burps abundantly, grungily snorts, and without telling me, binds me tight with a lasso of his tongue that stretches so long, mummifying my mind and mouth. I thought he was going to strangle me too,
but no! he just wanted to say: **"Shut up!"**

I love him…

11.

The Next Level

Immortality

Brenna reaches for the pill box. Fifteen pills a day, because
she has lost her way, people around her including her family
are not on her mindless level.
Brain cries FLY, to let it all go, the whole of her life has descended
so low, her self-worth torn, tattered, and emotionally shredded.
Her boys so young and insecure, she has hardly seen them, husband
phones the mental authority too regularly and admits her into hospital
care unnecessarily, using the institution as an escape for his lack of
understanding in how to help her. She does not wash, she eats too
much, three double chins and a pot belly, her nerves screwed up,
repeatedly, frenetically screaming at everyone and everything.
The scars of her father's behaviour, mirror her emotions.
She has inherited his personality traits. Something happened
she cannot recall; The big bad wolf has walked through her door,
and Hiss let him in, together they have hitched a plan,
it is time for Brenna to join their clan, they are both luring her in.

Where is her brother the one who is supposed to be always there?

He did not come back home because he found it a sad place to be,
he ventured out there, travelling about, cutting ties with his family.

Both parents and childhood pets Misty and Jesse have passed away.
Brenna feels unloved, she has new pets to care for, husband has found
hobbies for entertainment to escape her crazy moments.
Their marriage broken down ruined by the mental illness.
Brenna bakes a pill sponge cake, laced with alcohol too.
She eats it all when the children are asleep, washing it down with a
cocktail of drinks, then realising it is the wrong thing to do,
she phones an emergency counselling service *and passes out!*

Siren sounds, blue light flashes, the neighbours peering from behind
curtains, three police officer heroes rescue her in time. Medical staff in
the hospital pump the poisons out, she has no idea what is happening
right now.
The ambulance speed to a mental health place, she is heavily sleeping,
unaware of the panic around.

She wakes up next morning, in an empty room,
with a tiny, barred window. No bedding just a mattress, and naked.
Where are her clothes?
How did she get here?

"I carried you here!"

The hero Hiss whispers with a grin, while the wolf sniggers
behind his back saying,

"Party time Brenna, with me and him!"

12.

High Needs!

Sexual adventures

There is nothing to do in a lock up room,
the wolfs party idea is tempting, a bed and a mattress and a heavy oak
door, with a hatch that slides to view, the room is to keep a person safe
when their head spins gloom.
The Hiss curls himself around Brenna, flicking his tail at the wolf,
"She is mine!" he hisses at the feral foe; *"disappear now you fool!*
Her clothes neatly stacked at the bottom of the bed, she puts them on,
her thoughts a blank puzzle. The wolf howls and yowls gripping her
brain she wants to muzzle his nose to stop the sensitive sound pain.
She hears voices inside her mind telling her to look each way. They
beckon her to follow them, on either side of her brain. She holds her
head up and takes off her clothes again, to make a rope out of them,
she needs to escape out of the room.
The wolf snarls as he leaps on her back and
the Hiss spits at him to move,
she feels a bite at the nape and the wolf is rocking away.
Something uncomfortable presses against her behind, she realises what
the big bad wolf is doing, her arms flapping agitated backwards,
she punches the wolf's jaw. *"Let me out of here!"* she shouts aloud!

"I am trapped with two beasts today!"

The wolf clings on to her shoulders his paws around her neck,
his claws grasping her to sharp pain.
Brenna screams out, she can feel blood goo, trickling down her
shoulder blade. Her body tightens as the Hiss contracts in temper
squeezing the life out of her, he spits out venom at the feral foe who
loosens his grip and unexpectedly falls to the floor surrendering to the
poison then disappears out of view.
Brenna sobs huge tears shaking vigorously, pulling the Hiss away, her
mind does not know what to do next. Suffocating inside, feeling faint,
emotions out of control, her bare body writhes feverish with lust.
The door unlocks, a buxom nurse enters with porridge, a banana
and orange juice, she sees Brenna whimpering on the floor clutching
her stomach, tears flooding her face angrily moaning and groaning
on the floor.

"The wolf was trying to rape me, and the Hiss will not let him take me!"

It is a strange feeling to be delusional and sexually turned on
at same time.

*"There is no one here, my dear, put your clothes on young lady and have your
breakfast, take the medicine prescribed and go to sleep."*
The nurse casually says: *"You are hallucinating!"*

The Hiss slips away under the bed, the wolf has disappeared.

"Marry me!" the sneaky unusual reptile insists:
"Our journey has just begun"

Brenna's time in hospital is dragging on, so many issues and dramas within four whitewashed walls. When she feels low, she sees wild creatures in the carpet, lions, and tigers roaring, ready to leap, the Hiss is not scared he is lying at her feet, protecting her from wild feline aggravation.

Junior doctors are interested in her ill health. Pareidolia is a welcome subject, this imaginary hiss is a story of interest, Brenna is accommodating to talk things out, but she feels drained from the assessment chats.

"Shall I poison the doctors?" The Hiss does not like his queen to be anxious this makes him want to hunt and extinguish others. She does not hear him, she is heavily medicated, ranting in speech regularly, repeatedly, annoying the other patients' moods. The Hiss becomes upset that she is mind lost within, and decides it is time to human bin. He stalks and sniffs, feeling for fears, if his senses are threatened, the patient will die by his vile venom, or a slow strangulation while they lie in their bed. Hiss slithers into a room noticing two patients amorously nakedly playing, the nursing staff have not seen the passions running high as their bed rocks frenetically. Hiss smells sweaty warmth, he tastes blood through their skin, then whips out his tongue sucking them in whole into his mouth, bones crack bend and break, the couple scream in frightful despair, as faeces, vomit, and urine splatter everywhere, they are both crushed beyond repair, their blood draining out congealing everywhere, with stench so strongly putrid smelling of metal and raw.

Brenna senses something is happening and lethargically stumbles into the room to find her keeper.

Hiss lies in the bed with a mouth full of feet and entrails splattered on the white linen with human hair flying in the air.

"Oh my God! Hiss! What have you done? They were only loving each other,
this is wrong! Have you no shame? No instinct of morals? no remorse in hearing
pain? are you really this shallow? Do you enjoy the killing game?

Hiss opens his mouth and mangled feet drop to the floor, there's
nothing left of the other body parts and with a huge burp,
spits out angrily:

"I do not eat porridge"

He disappears into the utility room disappointed in Brenna's reaction.
She sighs, blinks her eyes, the surreal moment is gone, she mutters
"I feel sexy now!" stumbling into bed sleepily sedated, hoping
that the Hiss will go away permanently and find another person for
gatekeeper prey.

13.

The End of the Road

Relationship disasters

Brenna's marriage has ended, future relationships are worse, Hiss will not accept a man in her life, he demands she becomes his wife, or he will cause further mayhem with anyone she meets.

He fuels negativity, threatens to kill all in their way, an anti-social possessive creepy shadow creature, all Brenna's relationships constantly fail, she revolves in hallucination bubbles.

"I will not be your wife, you do not fully show yourself, and it will become bestiality. I am not like that!"

Hiss circles her, his wife to be, and tells her this is *all her fantasy.* She is the one who imagines things, he only looks after her with passion flaring from a visible eye. *"No! No! not at all!"* she stamps her feet in temper.

"I heard you in the park, you chose me, then followed me home and stayed!"

Hiss spits the ground and disappears thunderously belting his tail. There will not be any mutual agreement for now.

She lies in bed, images flooding her mind, hiss might be right? This is her fantasy land. She has no control over her sexual feelings they turn on over strange things in sound. Licking, paper rustling, scissors cutting, chocolate and sweet sucking, causing warm flushes to appear on her neck and cheeks, her love bush is firing up.

Unexpectedly Hiss appears and slides onto her stomach!

"You want me now my honey? Shall I nuzzle you?"

Brenna jolts herself out of a trance and stands up in a haste. *"Go away!"*

She elbows the Hiss to the ground then kicks him out of the way.

Hiss braces himself higher, a sizzling black spit slur foaming his mouth,

he is going to strike her, then backs down, realising his beloved is

attacking him with lost senses. *"I will return when you have calmed down!"*

He hisses a gruff; ***"Goodbye my love, for now!"***

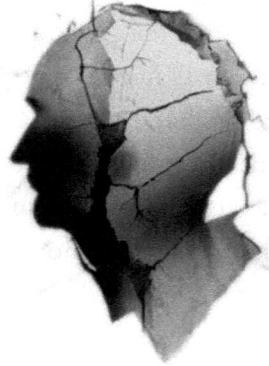

14.

Nightmares

Relationship misjudgement

Hiss adapts to Brenna's new relationships with negative relish, she enters a relationship with a man who overindulges in alcohol, and constantly drinks to oblivion. Her judgement of friendships and people's characters seem impulsively poor, she must like to be challenged. It is hard to live with someone who has no respect while intoxicated, and who is selfish with lack of care. A hiss relative occupies his mind, with a hoard of invisible monsters who feed off his volatile outbursts.

The air in the house fraught from verbal fights of her partners late nights out, his monster clan encouraging Brenna's relationship to severe. Brenna cannot shake his creature thoughts off her back, and with her partner struggling with hiss, demons of his own, their love will never last.

She saw the Angel of Darkness one night, its shadow sheltering her from a violent night of domestic attack, her eyes badly bruised, her relatives do not want to get involved, why doesn't her guardian Hiss protect her soul? Where is he? when she needs him? He is too busy birthing an army of hidden zombies in her partner's sad mind. Heavy energy waves swamp the house, she is living in fear of a man with little empathy for her happiness.

Will she ever have a normal life? she feels constantly threatened, insecure, on edge, and family members have no idea how dangerous a drinking cohabiting relation can be in, no one cares, they really **do not care!**
No one sees it happening. Ignorance is a sad virtue.
Why do people not understand substance addiction? it's a lifelong curse?
They show no feelings of empathy or sympathy and make her domestic situations worse. Brenna is hopelessly lost, her 'will' is decaying.
Family members say, *"You have to talk and make things work"*.
If people only knew the danger seeping in and ruining lives and the brute partner does not care, causing further heartache and home damage. A broken glass door, a phone smashed, a throat grab, and so many nights broken hearted in floods of tears. Thrown out of the house on New Year Eve, in freezing frost and ice on the ground with barely any clothes to keep warm, while baby squalls and he her second partner is oblivious to all.
Why did he get involved with her if he will never change his habits?
There is a new birth in this unsettled unhappy home, and:

it is not Jesus for sure!

Hiss duplicates another hiss brother to molest minds and worry her even more. It is amazing how a mythical creature can multiply in a cloud of meddling disruption causing issues to infest and brew.
How she puts up with darkness masking a family home with children growing insecure? lightning striking heavy chest pains, frightening her confused mind into a curdled beaten mess. She feels frail, exhausted, and worn.

She calls time on the insensitive troubled man, who has no understanding of good parenting unless it came off a pub pump. She leaves him and finds a new home to raise the children on her own, hoping to leave her guardian Hiss behind with the unpredictable ex to screw his mind, it's not to be, as all the hiss menageries are stuck on her, *determined to secure her as their own.*

She hopes a new life will reap in a new love who will devote himself more, but hissing shadow monsters insist sleeping in her bed, cuddling her back, and snogging her ears from behind, while her marital hiss nestles between her legs, warming her crotch every night.

She is lonely her mental state is high. She cringes sexual pain, chews pillow ends, as sexual irritation explodes on fire, erupting orgasmic larva overflows and sensual desires. Her high is a volcanic surge of electrical energy, firing explosive sensuality.

She breaks down into a fantasy mess escaping from the relationship has taken its toll. Brenna resides in a psychiatric ward again, same people, same show.

The brute ex-lover looks after the children until she recovers.

She lies under sedation, sectioned within mental health walls for a month, until the madness subsides again.

Hiss rejoices he has more killing choices, stalking human mixed weak emotions from oblivious patients.

A young anorexic girl in the mental health ward does not belong there, but there is no bed space in other hospitals to send her elsewhere.

Her eating habits in decline, the Hiss, and his family of abusive reptiles, spit poison in her mouth until the young lady chokes and dies.

If she does not like eating, they like human food....

and young girls taste nice.

Is Hiss immortal? Or does he eventually go away?
If she could see her surreal allies, she would find a way to rid them,
but they float in her distorted confused mind.
Shame! Madness survives throughout time!

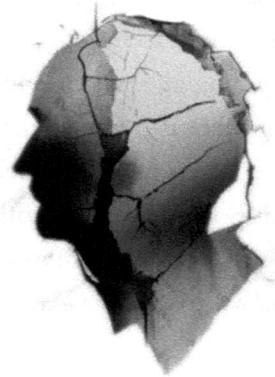

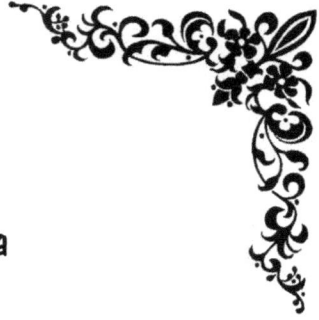

15.
Poem for Brenna
Home

My future was gone the true love
had lasted too long. New reality
fractious mood,
Finding it hard to find the good
Born again into the wild
Forever an abandoned child
Forgiveness, justice, regrets
Time passes I must forget.
The roots were poison
Infecting our reason, I wanted everything
In every season I spared no expense
Not to my feelings. My fortitude,
my friends. My energy knew no end
But now I am home in bliss
And with my own
All snuggled and not alone
A sonsie lass again running
and laughing, In the rain, overcoming loss and pain.
Illusion turns to disillusion I can only gain.

By *Anne-Louise Lowrey* author of
"Now looking back going forward, a journey of well being through Schizophrenia" and
"My Schizo-Affective Garden of Eden."

16.

Single-Parent Living Within: The Head Maze - Confusion

Going it alone with children in tow.

Looking around the empty house, Brenna feels a huge gut loss.

She has never been on her own, bills always paid by previous husband,
her friend kindly donated basic furniture, and organised a carpet to
for the living room, then with a wave she tells her:
"That is all, I am leaving you to sort yourself out,
this has drained me to help you."
The children are young, so vulnerable, and confused.
"This is not a holiday!" the 4 years of age son says.
He recognises the town where they regularly travelled to shop,
Brenna feels guilty she made things up to take them away from
their father from a situation that was dangerously rough.
She 'group' hugs the children and looks at the bags piled up,
There is so much to do to sort the children's needs.
A new school, make the home comfortable, find activities,
for the kids to do, she switches off the phone for weeks,
to think, to plan, and build stability for her children,
this is all new to her and responsibility scary.

The last thing the brute said was that she will never cope,
But the Hiss intervened and said, *"Let him go!"* so she did,
as she knew her partner would have reaped hazard from the
poisonous fluid his throat flowed.
"I can do this I can!" she silently vows...
not realising that there would be no support for her emotions,
from relatives, it is too late to go back to him now.
How does her head think? She begins her new task, as mother and
father in one to her children, will she cope? will her guardianship last?
Will she end up inside mental health sanctuary and her children will
disperse? to other people for home care, knowing that she will not see
them again, until they are older to meet her on their own?
"I can do this! I can!" her head screams out again!
"But I am fuddled in a haze, and no idea what route to take?"
Her brain is triggering within her in all sorts of ways.
Hiss appears sliding up her spine, she curdles a silent scream as he
tickles her back, the children are upstairs they have a routine time for
bed, so, he sits on her lap and makes plans for her mind.
*"You will become a queen and serve men; they may help you
or want only an intimate gain; this will keep you stable
if you play the fantasy game"*
Hiss snuggles her ear his tongue dips in and out, she feels a choking
sensation in her gullet and her lips glisten wet when he wraps his long
body around, his tail slithers in her mouth as he prods her to suck,
like a baby bewildered her mind feels sexually muddled and brain-fog
rough. Flashes of light glimmer through her eyes, as tinkles of bells
ring all around, she hopes the soft rings are angels guarding her soul, to
stop the demons of her mind gaining control.

"I will protect my children, I will, I will,
I will never think of demonic words like suffocate and kill!"
She is washing crockery in a basin of suds, and hears a large crack
a wine glass smashes fragments of shard, her brain is strong
so powerful so intent, but yearns to do wrong, dual personality and
super sense qualities, have heightened inside her head.
"I can cope with this single parenthood with my lovely three.
I will let my path flow and accept men who will betroth to me!"
The angels are all around, they ship, and they shape, they are from
the dark side, and they are from the light, and there's fairy's in-between
to meddle things right. The vibes in the air electrify her mind, lines
in front of her eyes are speeding past, her head is one way her arms
another, her legs feel heavy then run after each other.
"I can do this!" she repeats over, and over, again, her heart beating fast
as she knows if she collapsed her demons spill out.
Hiss will devour her children, or a monster within her thirsting for
death will grab her in a black moment of frenzies, leave her with
shame, a ruined life,
her children blood drained and soul drowned.
"I can do this I can do this!" her 'will' repeats over, and over, again.
The road ahead is 15 years long, her life consumed in child's play, keep
them active, keep them fit, iron each crease that springs hate their way,
there are emotions of clashes that keep attacking with venom and spite,
but it is all invisible air. It is possible to push air along, diffuse negativity
and apologise for hurting and misguidance, at each stage of life. It
doesn't help that her sex nerves are astray, no man in the moment to
help her on her way, to an orgasmic blast and a fainting fit, of high
emotion a flowing ambience of need, to calm the head like a dopamine

fill, because hers is full of sexual need to adjust her head in coping with all, so no one should belittle, or woman call, when chemical imbalance *is the root of it all!*

"I am not a slag. Or a whore!
It is up to me if I want men at my door, to help with my needs.
I can hear the whispers out there, the gossipers stare,
witch-crafting soul-stabbing my demise!"

With sorrow she thinks deeply inside her soul, as a candle is flickering low, snug in her bed as the light hangs low, the children seem to realise not to be naughty, as mummy is sick, but their security is at risk, who wants to live with strangers because mum is amiss? Brenna is lucky her kids aged 6, 4 and 2, seem to sense her illness and stay quiet and good. Thankyou Angels who helped them to be mindfully, misunderstood, and ignorant to her well-being health needs.

The Head Maze – Panic!

Confusion leads to panic, isolation, and state of oblivion.
The maze in the mind is becoming a dread, everything I see
I read misread, the connections, the links, are in my face,
but when I follow them, I walk through a maze, constantly
tripping, losing myself, heart fluttering with ill ease.
I see random insects, spiders and bees crawling on me but then
I gasp, and they disappear like a blown-up fantasy.
I gabble, I chat, I fall in love so many times, but no one wants
me when my moods arise. I start to run around in bursts of panic
the A.D.H.D kicks in, I fall depressed, gabbling, moody,
aggressively obsessed.

I rant and rave throw pots away, slamming doors so hard
they become loose,
I swear and cuss even though no-ones there, raucously loud and rude.
The neighbours call the police, because of the volatile sounds.
"Hello officer, can I help you!?" I say, in the sweetest voice.
They go away after inspecting the children when I have not done
anything incriminating at all! Off course the children have an unsettled
life, and the Hiss encourages me to be sexual, he nestles and slides
along my crotch at night to heighten my tingling buds and tells me to
reach for the phone to call a lonely soul, but at least the children do
not have a stepdad, who shouts! Or causes domestic arguing issues to
unsettle their life!
"Are you talking about me?" Hiss gurgles flicking his tail ferociously,
he can read my mind so quickly *"Hiss! you do stir my emotions!*
You lip slide me with your forked tongue and fear my love nest
with your poison spats!" I become flustered and nervous, waving my arms
about, angrily staring the Hiss out! but he's still a mist with body bits.
"I thought you liked a tickle?" Hiss rasps with a gruff, then slinks away
under the sofa, to escape my frenetic rising temper. *"Shhhh!"* he lisps
settling for sleep.

17.

Lonely Living

My mind is madness, delusional feelings, emotionally euphoric,
how can I control sexuality? During a mania attack?
If I ask for a pill the emotions die down, but then slumber
hits me deeply and I cannot awaken easily. Why should I lose the
opportunity to love while living? just because the mind has its own path
and confuses my being?
No one understands the mind waves are uncontrollable, the fastness
of thought patterns surpasses the body's ability to keep up, distorting
vision and mobility.
I try to settle with people as lovers, but my personal space feels
violated, and possessiveness is rife. It feels like riding a bike with the
legs dangling out, the bike seat rubs, and I sweat and shake. The heat
revs up with energy sparks, my face becomes rosy and dark, the love
lips pump up with fleshy itching need.
Fantasies in the mind to feed the bipolar high pain, needs lots of sex,
or give it up. When desire is unfulfilled the irritation fills my throat, a
horny throttled larynx vibrates a rough gurgling sound. Simultaneous
quivering luscious lips rocking my pelvic boat. Abusive words scream
out! Veins fill the blood stream with bursting ripples, the body shakes,
and legs run around, everything in the home breaks,
as mind thoughts spill libido, and aggressive behaviour overtakes.
Who wants to be a partner when this destructive attitude is rife?

People are not human machinery or robots, and I do not know how to love gently.

Normally sexual need can start and stop at will, but not in high mood swing rhythms, once the plug of energy ignites the sexual battle commences, the more heat conjures, the more menacing the advances, this pushes partners away, they go and not come back, and leaves a lonely mess to sort myself out.

Life is lonely when the Hiss is 'hissing sizzling' the back of my head, tickling my pink fancy encouraging adventure in someone else's bed. The children are powerless they have no clue, why mummy changes partners and breaks her own heart too, they scarper when they hear the hysterical screaming from broken relationships, and disappear into their rooms finding something to do, hoping mothers broken crazy moods go away. My children's daily life is miserable often.

Hiss is silently stalking in the shadows, waiting for the moment when the children are asleep, he has found another mysterious friend to bother me.

Hiss spits and spats; *"Hello! my bride to be, a visitor has arrived for pumpkins and crumpets. Welcome him please!"* another beady eye peers from a shrouded mist.

A slurp and spit, another poison fuelled tongue darting about, no body, just a spitting fired up sigh. Hiss and his mates always appear when I am lying down at my lowest ebb, exhausted from the daily chores.

My groin stirs, an arousal kicks within, the hiss wraps me tightly as I lay with head sin. My right leg is itchy, crawling feelings arise the invisible tongue works itself through my trousers to my luscious surprise. I sweat, shudder and shake.

I know I need to break away, my heart is pained dull and lonely, I scare people away, the Hiss and his friends seem imaginatively phoney.

"No! No! No!" I shout. *"Go away you volatile creatures!"*

I reach for pills and swallow them fast, soon, I am dozing,
hiss and friends can play somewhere else. How much longer will
fantasies fill my head?
From a corner at the top of my crown, Satan sits there swishing his
tail with a leery frown. The sensations are pleasurable when high as a
kite, but visions can be a terrifying sight. I have learnt not be afraid,
to embrace every high wave, and to realise I am a different sort of
human being, but no one understands my sexual meaning, as gnawing
pains of negativity stab me below, and once again anger I show, with
hotwired nerves racing my pulse, I am sure there are others suffering
a hot bodied fuse. My dear friend has written again a spirited poem,
so I do not feel ashamed. She suffers too with different visitors of her
own, everyone has issues but sometimes the inner sin never shows, bad
luck for those of us who are open minded to invite madness to dinner,
with the taste of blood as jam in a sandwich, dreaming obliviously of a
poisoned cup of green tea.

18.

The Heart

By *Anne-Louise Lowrey (author)*

The sun shone like a heartbreak
Stark and unforgiving
The sky was
The kind of bright blue
That a child would paint
Yet, there was no comfort
No prayerful saint
The dandelions pushed
Through the cracks
In the paving
But nothing could quell my craving
The birds, twittered
Cackled and crowed
The weather was clement
But last week it snowed
I couldn't see the beauty
Relentlessly pursued by duty
I'd die if I couldn't love, cry out in pain
Nothing would be the same
The heart survives, torn and tough
Sometimes bleeding
Bruised and rough
Try praying, or meditating
Or searching your soul
Believe you are enough.

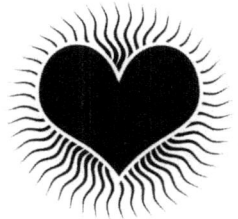

19.

Finding My Inner Self

"*I cannot go on like this!*"
I lie in bed painting mind circles in the yellowing flaking Artex ceiling,
"*I have to let the Hiss family go but I don't know how?*"
The bed covers move and lift, and a cold breeze
blows between my legs, I feel a kiss on my cherry lips.
I scream. "*Get off me Hiss!*"
A beady eye appears next to me within silver misty sparkles,
and a lisping tongue snuffles a deep low sound.
"*I am here next to you! and so am I!*" a second voice whispers.
I look under the covers, and no one is there, I am living through
another psychosis lost thought, the pills do not work
I have too many issues, muddling in brain delusion and senses buzzed
in a nondescript way.
I see a grey shadow behind the curtain, my eyes dance shape changes,
and the grey shadows swiftly adapt a different form,
I feel depressed and forlorn as I stare at the pills on my bed side table,
deciding whether to take them all. The walls are coming closer
the ceiling is closing in,
the air is getting tighter, my breathing is shallow and thin.
Who will collect my youngest from nursery? the other two will feel
abandoned at school, this is not a good moment, for me to leave for
ever, the children will become monster doomed!
A drooping flower has a chance to rise if watered again,
and so does the soul.

One must set small goals of happiness achievement and nourish the inner self. Finding the right things to do to stop the pressured view of an externally cruel world is not easy but having a selfless act of understanding that one can be toxic to others if they do not balance the good and bad, will save others from going mad.

The secret is the power of the "will" held within the soul.

Power to feel well. Power to feel good. Power to avoid negativity and power to physically move. Power to feel love from beautiful music, to breathe in nature and creative sights. Power to realise that everything will unfold right. There is a way to fight through a brick head, there is a light at the end of the tunnel if one believes in themselves and loves their inner self.

Society is constantly visually needy with controlling high tech spies confusing thought patterns to follow a life path of unsuitability. Like lambs to the slaughter brainwashed in opaqueness with battered soulless spirit. People live in pockets of wide energy barriers within hazy clouded minds, sunken and depressed. Strangers show sympathy but forget to have empathy.

Sympathy is a get out clause to evade responsibility towards another, so no help to the suffering this way and the 'ill' smother. Having empathy is comforting and rewarding because someone will put themselves out to help another move towards a better life. Empathy is an involvement it takes up time to show one cares, unfortunately in society not all want to be available for others out there.

The culprit is ignorance, ignorance to feel the destructive emotions of those who need help,

and how a person can live their 'sorted' cushioned life without feeling guilt for others is unbelievable within, itself.

Hiss feeds off those who are vulnerably weak causing mayhem and emotional disturbance, he pounces to devour their 'mind' for dinners and treats.

There is power that everyone owns if they unlock their inner gifts and purpose.

A hobby or work undiscovered, or a physical talent unexplored, or doing good for others as worthy causes, or explore by learning knowledge through educating themself. Life is for living but living should also be giving support to the lonely and destitute who are too weak to find their way. More understanding of humanity needs can help to prevent a tormenting Hiss or the wolf, from knocking on a disturbed mind door.

There is a lurking third mind creature, a hissing spitting monster who feeds of grandeur power controlling human minds which he cannot resist. No one is better than any-one else, so escape if cornered this way by someone possessed, or their victim soul will be a prisoner entwined in their deceptive psychotic pitted mind.

Everybody journeys differently and true spirit is not in wealth, at the end of physical life living, money and objects are worthless eternally, because the soul will move on independently by itself.

20.

Power

By *Anne-Louise Lowrey (author)*

Surrender no more
Time to arrive on the shore
Clamber over the stones
Face life alone
Rigid principles
Die without sense or reason
No room for mistakes
No falsehoods, treason
The cycle of life
Ever present
I worked on the allotment
The weather was pleasant
I found out that the rain
Was as great as sunshine
And darkness was a time for rest
The past is still with me
It is a difficult test
Now, I speak freely
Open hearts open mind
Special forces, trying hard to be kind
There's no future in vengeance
No need to be bitter
There's a faint resemblance
Of gold to glitter
One World One love
Joy of life reigns from above

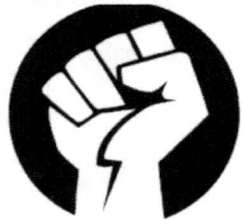

21.

Living Life Moves On

Why dark thoughts?

The children have grown, I live on my own, I reap what I sow, life has not been good to me, but when my mind is in torment how can a person reason with oneself? I am a fuddle, a brain wave muddle? What will I do with myself? I do not get on with people they suffocate my thoughts, so much lying and deceiving has anyone spared a thought? Corrupting stirring from others ignite poor mental health, and if it's not the wolf in sheep's clothing attacking, it's the Hiss stalking myself. Outer influences bring out vile sin, but in a court of judgement can a person distinguish a good or bad soul? My head tells me to stop thinking of 'ill doings' towards others, but when people show their dark side outside in, the psychosis within me flares up, and I mind blow up. I emulate other peoples' thoughts.

Abusive shouting words spill out of my tongue. I know this is wrong. The world is a large mirror bouncing off others around, humans are clones of themselves acting scenarios causing conflict and fight.

An ability to feel and see beyond others is like meeting hell and heaven as one, but if someone makes a poor move in the wrong direction, the wolf, and the Hiss spring from fuzzy brain fog. Who knows who pulls the string of visions? From above?

It is something from energy, darkness, and light, and it is empathy that makes up the difference, unfortunately humans have not got this right. Death by self-infliction might happen and people can avoid it, by feeling love for the soul inside. Eyes are treacherous in those who are born from dark energy, but no one else notices, because there is too much focus on human body, not enough attention to spirit and soul, it is easy to see a gloomy character, one who will never change, but there seems to be ignorance in masses of human's brains.

So why do things go wrong in the world? is it because people *like* how they feel? they feed of pleasurable instinct, and instinct can swing positive in love, or negative to kill. The power of the gut is the heart of all movement, and the choices one makes, but people are gaslighted during their life path journey, to function their brains in a certain *following way!'* so the wolf and the Hiss feed of unstable minds, twisting humans to change what they think, do, or say.

The Hunger Games are born from this life pathway from human mind monsters and demons within having conflicts living each day. Light plays tricks on humanity, it really confuses the brain, constant changes of weather also cause havoc this way.

22.

The FINAL One For Me?

She lies sunbathing in the warm, hoping the Hiss is tanning elsewhere.
This moment in time there is peace in her mind, no visions,
no sounds, no stares. A man pops his head over the fence,
his face looks friendly and kind-hearted, her heart skips a beat,
when he speaks, his voice is cute quirky sounding.
"Hello gorgeous!" he winks, while eyeing her ample breasts,
she feels a little uncomfortable, it's been a while since meeting
the other sex.
"Weather is great today, fancy a drink later in a cosy place?"
He hopes she will say yes.
She thinks for a minute wondering if it is worth it, relationships have
been destructive before, and she knows the Hiss will not like it, and the
wolf will creep in like before. He seems kind though and it is summer,
company is nice in lighter long days.
His age is ten years older so surely? he might be the one? and grateful
to be in her life?
"Ok" she warily answers *"We can meet in the pub near the canal"*
One drink and chat will not cause damage to her soul, she thinks
deeply, she doesn't want her heart broken again.
In the evening she looks 'pretty and wild' he cannot believe she said
yes, by the end of the night he says she looks beautiful in the flimsy
pink spotted dress.

She should have known not to fall so quickly, but loneliness is an insecure thing, a gentle aged man like he, surely will feel heaven blessed, he cannot be a threat to her *surely?*

She walks with him to his house for coffee, insisting they are only platonic friends. He tells her this will be ok for now, then shocks her with the next words he said.

"I have mental health issues I hope you can see beyond that"

She is a little disappointed as his health seemed to mirror hers. Maybe he is her twin flame? and they both can work out their differences together?

"If it doesn't work out with him, it won't work with anyone!" she bites her lips and twiddles her hair in frustration but decides to give it a chance, she has desires of love and nurturing towards him, sensing his sadness inside.

A friend once said to her if she meets a man whose eyebrows meet close together, they hide personality issues within, so why didn't she take her friends advice and withdrew from the friendship before problems start to begin?

They suffer heated characters clashes head on! Like mirrors of each other, she has a short fuse in temper because he twists things about, saying he is doing something else then changes his plans around. He seems to be narcissistic, but she behaves that way as well. Whatever she says, whatever she does, he makes sure she feels *guilty as hell.* She sees the dark shadow hanging on his back it was intimidating looking, needy, and bad.

A large grey monster, a heavy powerful 'mind beast' who twists every conversation they have. She notices strange things about him, he can change energy vibes in the air, mind reading her thoughts to make her believe that she instigates every domestic argument they share. He diverts his mind in daily tasks, she never knows where she stands with him, he is difficult to please in bed, and never takes the love lead which drains her health day to day.

His blue eyes magnetise hers drawing her into a daze. Hiss is incredibly angry because she pushes him away, and the wolf does not appear he never shows his face, perhaps the monster hanging onto to her lovers back has taken the wolfs place? a snake appears in her lovers eyes every time he becomes sombre or confused, his luring blue view hardened a gaze, no flickers of love in them.

He is an infectious character she found hard to let go and move on, he seems to be needy to buy attention, rather than desire her as the only one. She feels she is a temporary duvet cover while he hides his real feelings elsewhere. She breaks up with him so many times he retreats into his shell inventing controlling moves deep in his mind with an icy stone glare, hooking up with other woman with different monsters as his best friend. Every time they break up, they go back to each other over, and over, again. She is convinced he is part of her soul, embedded deeply within hers, she vows to conquer all the evils they hold inside their consciousness, to bring peace to their troubled brains, he's an awkward man who never sees the errors of his ways. A difficult man to be with, this relationship looks doomed again.

23.

Monsters Within

Demons hide skulking under the bed, others hide in the head,
creating a stigma in people with unbalanced thoughts.
Whispers appear whenever I am near because people fear the power
of an unusual mind. Why should I apologise? for the monsters
passing through? because the dark clouds ascending over my intuitive
mind, try to save me from thoughtless humankind. I meditate and pray
negative thoughts away, realising wickedness mind grows carelessly,
because people build dark toxicity from environment and other
humans' actions, causing lucid crazed thoughts to be bred.
Death is not the greatest loss in life, it is the sadness dying inside the
soul while living.
We give and we take, and we take, and we give, it is not a faultless,
smooth ride this surreal world of sin, cruelty and unforgiving.
I will not apologise for the demons within me because no one
apologises for witnessing me this way, they do not understand the
power it takes to make the monsters inside my head to run away.
They sinisterly crawl back in through another chameleon disguise,
visually showing through psychotic eyes. This can happen to anyone,
at any time, a trigger of emotional instability, their persona curtain
falls away with a negative slump and a loss of power to control head
thoughts mangled deep.
Too many personality disorders in one mind will cause multiple issues,

there is no excuse to behave ill within will, but if hell is in the eye
of the beholders' soul, do the eyes need gouging? to cast evil aside?
Satan lays waiting within other humans too? inflicting wounds of
hurtful scars in brainwaves causing disarray amongst the whole
of humanity.
So what? If I am a beast? I will bury the angry pain with my smile.
All people walk a unique life path, but the windows of our soul show
everyone their true colours, the Universe will judge, when it is time for
each of us to fall.

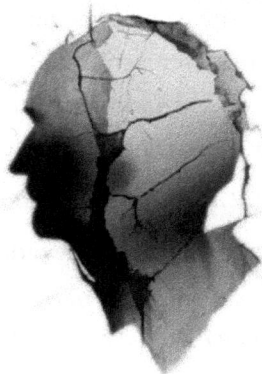

24.
Zombified

He jumbles her so much in mincing his words she begins to feel she cannot control her own life. Her urges to visit him are unnatural, drawn into a lion's den he has eaten her heart and caged her mind. She sits on the bench her green eyes dulled, while pictures in the clouds show fighting scenes above, she is desperate to relieve her trapped thoughts.

She has a need to cling onto her lover who's sting has bitten her to be pleasing his every whim. She focuses on loving him, she cannot understand why he has taken her nurturing for granted, she cannot comprehend why he is never happy, the huge grey monster breathing more spirited poisonous clouds onto him.

She sees a dark shadow in the corner of his room, a black shape of a figure, or maybe it is his alto ego? which ships and shapes between dual personality that he projects, pouring misery into both of their souls. A crackle a spit, a thump on the bed and the Hiss has re-entered the game, overcasting her partner, he has had enough of watching the doomed friendship, pumping up his venom to senselessly knock him out. Hiss wants Brenna, his bride back!

"It's taken you a long time to rescue me, where were you?"

I am gratefully relieved.

"I was here all the time watching you go crazily insane!
His dual headed monster is not the best enemy to fight!"

The Hiss informs me with knowledge of my lovers' personality
disorder I never knew he had. I exhaustedly reply:

*"Better late than never! Let's go home
I will end the relationship for ever this time."*

Hiss whispers a patronising sneer,

"Are you seeing sensibly now? My bride to be friend?"

"Yes" I hesitantly answer with driven positivity, *but deep down I am not sure
at all!*

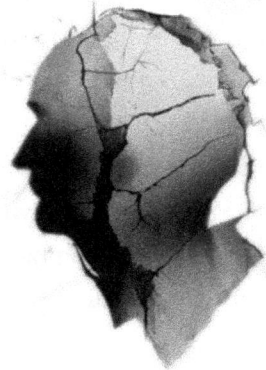

25.

Godly Snake Charming World

The world is in chaos from negative thought,
built on heavy atmosphere and torrid rain pours.
The philosophy scholars wrote history to suit themselves
as centuries rolled over in change. Humankind slaughtered world-wide
as time entered new decades, but for what noble cause?
To seek superiority? Instead of love? to seek gold that turns to dust.
To rampage and taste the flesh of nubile skin?
deaden the body and digging a hole to bin,
then hypocritically pray to the mighty one above without remorse?
Who said it was one God who dominated the Universe?

When all living people can be gods within themselves unlocking their
true worth. Create magic, cast a spell, enhance their senses to do good
for all.

Energy is the source that has power, to ship shape, change, helping
living beings become strong, create sadness, badness, hatred for others,
kindness, benevolence, love for one another.

Energy is a powerful source.

Now the gods of old are here to sort the mess, history of all has
replenished again, playing rhythm through human ears, snake charming
hypnosis, banishing psychosis, and clearing darkness of evil doing,
enlightening souls a clear view of heaven in colours of warmth with
brightness of a new happy dawn.

The planets are in line now the celestials can recycle each person who is born, who begins as dust and progresses to womb birth, and those that turn to dust after death occurs, are returning as angels in forms of mist and light, to sprinkle their magic and healing consciousness while people sleep, so on awakening they change their steadfast belief. Living the new revolving surreal Earth stage, where delusion has split into modern dimensions, the old world in one, the new one in another. Rhythm is the snake charmer, and everyone is in line to pass the test of staying alive. To find their goal the reason for birth and return to energy when their time as dispersed. For those set fast in thickness and dim, they will renew back into the world of sin, but those who heal and realise their talent, a new world is forming as the planets revolve balanced. Numbers, equations, energy formations, the secret of eternal life has always been here, there is no one superior only light the energy powerful force, it's the belief in a devil snake who has ruled everyone unclean. History muddled in deceit and painted in lies, washed over, ignored, within everyone's blind eyes. Generations of parents receive brainwash news, repeating the education over again, The Illuminati rules those trapped in ignorance.

A young child is vulnerable and sucked in, to this web of falsity and sin. Authorities educating to forget the true meaning of genetic heritage from the beginning of time.

The body hoodwinked but everyone's genes never lie.

A mask of dominant metricity shrouds the evolution of every ethnicity in the world, the eyes of every soul are now worth more than gold. Holding information of truth that needs telling. The snake is the one who started this mess, man fearing the creature and history spanned the rest.

The rhythm charmer and the celestials counting all in the birthing game, especially ones who can use their senses in exemplary psychic ways.

Life now evolves as a circle of truth, then dying and living again, the illuminati are the gods of intelligence who are throwing the dice of hungry destroying games.

We are all alien in a divided future which is torn in different energy dimensions serving human clones mirroring imaging infinity over again. Worn disillusioned life forms living in a fragmented fragile world, which doesn't really exist, we create our own illusions by ignorance and lack of faith within, but truth can release from within the enlightened spirit. Self-belief is the most valuable tool, because only yourself is the one who can progress, forget what's happening to the rest. Play the game by your own rules.

Governing forces cause each imprisoned mind to weave and turn walking this universe blind. They are like reptiles who slither and slide, charm whistling the frequency tune to mesmerise all who are not in tune to the changes in society.

Meditation is the key to execute the consciousness to relax by peaceful thinking, happy music, calming body. This encourages the will and soul within to lift and raise the veil of the sacred third eye that all possess. The pineal gland is the eternal chalice, where the chemicals release in the brain, and then in time controlling tyranny will fall. Consciousness will rise while alive, delusions will be clarity seen, but everyone is living through their own dreams, and only need to listen to themselves, not succumb bewitched by others means.

Love those who cross the same road but don't allow oneself to be trapped in organised thoughts. As the path to freeing the soul is a self-invested life pattern journey from beginning to end. Humans are born old souls, to live time out again until their soul rises to a new level of energy power, then they can claim to be eternal gods to live different life patterns again.

The hierarchy breed lies, the snake charmers heal lives, a snake will shed its skin and in the new world will eternally rise.

What has happened to the apple of knowledge? An apple is a fruit to enjoy not used as a tool for fearing, and if the children in the garden of Eden listened to their own pure soul, history would not have bred hatred in any shaped way, because a soul birth is pure and does not understand differences.

It is confusion which stems from double standard education, listening to diverse sources of contradictory information, that inherit confusing minds throughout a whole lifespan.

God and the Devil is within oneself, the dark and light side of us all. The snake creature is not the devil in disguise it is a reptile who can re-energise its skin for new growth, life lessons learned in an old world are defunct, and new-born life begins

In a new world of truth

67

26.

The Last Say...

I didn't think this will happen I truly did not think it would. My ex and I bounce off each other so badly it floods our senses with toxic fumes. He made up scenarios that weren't there, I became a ghostly figure with a frozen iced stare. We needed to go into the care unit, we both needed to stay, he one end of the corridor and I at the rear of the building with the communal room in the middle.

Both of us staring each out every day.

He sits hunched and mumbling, his eyes filled with dopey stuff,

I was sleeping, deeply oblivious to others who looked on. Now I have woken up.

He is lucky to have a caring family, he has visitors every day, but I just look out of the window counting the days my children will visit again. It is particularly important to have family support, but most people cannot deal with mental poor health. It frightens them to see their loved ones out of sorts emotionally, it's like witnessing the darkness of demonic hell.

At this moment of time, we both are too preoccupied in the tunnel of lost hope, to even know our relationship ever existed, and we are unaware what is happening in the psychiatric unit we stay in, too distracted in our own head mess to see

a woman screaming from four beds away. She awoke my heart with a thump, like a car being jumpstarted with leads I flung out of bed mind dazed. I look over to her and see worms crawling out of her blooded belly, with nits in her matted hair jumping into her eyes and mouth, as her tongue hangs parched fluffy and smelly.

"Nurse! Nurse!" I shout in bewilderment, my eyes darting distorted and wild. *"The lady near me is in distress!"*

No-one is here to sort the lady's troubled mind, blood keeps spilling on the floor, congealing into a brown fudge patch.

Are we abandoned? is there any nursing staff in this dingy old musty cold place?

It breathes a sadness of ill-doing and disgrace.

A young man walks into the room, bony and thin, his eyes sunken within. His lips misshapen severely, his face crooked to one side, he mutters and groans waving his hands around in circles then falls in a heap on the floor showing profound blue patches around his frow and jawline.

"Nurse! Nurse!" I shout once more. *"Fetch the doctors and security guards, bring other medical people if you can? Something is happening to these patients!"*

My heart pounds, my pulses beat terrified inside, but no one comes, so where are they? Am I abandoned for ever here as a recluse never found?

A doctor crawls through the door on his hands and knees, his ligaments torn and an arm missing, his stethoscope tied round his neck with eyes bulging, gasping for air. He collapses in front of the lady patient who is bleeding to death, and the thin-boned man who stabbed himself with a knife that he found in the nursing staff room.

What is happening? I have no idea, is my mind exploding fantasy fear? Is the medication an unsuitable pill? for me to witness such tragedy and a loss of people's *lives* and *will?*

The doors fly open a food trolley rolls in, the support worker delivering evening meals, mouth gagged with a tea cloth, lying on the trolley her arms and legs flailing, a spoon handle in her throat which throttles her larynx so tight she cannot cry. She's held down by the trolley handles with curtain pulls tying her wrists, her bones broken and bent, what did this lady do? to deserve all of this? are the meals that bad?

Who will stop all this trauma happening today?

The stench of blood, the people's faeces splatter, the bodies lying there, my gut spasms, I throw up spew shivering with fear, who is in the building?

Along the corridors I hear a commotion, heavy feet scuffing their heels along the shiny flooring, anger, aggressiveness, pained moans and wailing calls.

What is happening? with confused anxiety I hide under a table, then bursting through the door spill out nursing staff including doctors, with bitten deformed faces, bulging bloodied eyes, and broken mouths. Their eyes like glass staring soulless I am witnessing drugged up medical **ZOMBIES!** their hands holding sharp tools, attempting to slice each other as they staggered into the room *obliviously*. Gruesome curdling screams pitifully howl in the distance, I don't know what to do, where is the hiss to protect me? My soul screams fearfully inside.

"I am here!" Hiss growls in my ear: ***"Enjoy the gruesome ride!"***

Stomping monster creature army appear in purple smoke munching, crunching nursing staff in their ferocious mouth. A deformed lizard, a scaly bulbous snake, a large poisonous toad with three legs, a dragon big and strong, and a serpent so long and the biggest one of them all, a Komodo dragon smashing doors, his long tongue darting in and out spitting venom all around. I can see behind the creatures, trails of entrails from broken dead people, every-one is dead apart from me, and where is my partner? *"Where on earth is he?"*

"Oh Shit! I'm done. I thought you loved me Hiss!" I scream a nervous traumatised wail. I am rooted in paralysis shock as the huge Komodo dragon staring at me is bracing himself to swallow me whole. Will my hiss hero defend me, rescue me? or not at all? The Komodo curls out his tongue swiftly and I feel a splat of vomited sick.

I roll over in agony searing burning pains scorch my cheek. Hiss curls around my body gently snuffing a breeze in my tangled hair:

"Say that you will marry me, and the disillusions will disappear!"

he urgently requests approval and commitment. With a weak voice and crushed body, I pitifully splutter:

"Burn in Hell! Burn! I do not marry figments of my imagination!

The Komodo dragon unexpectedly disappears, the Hiss and monster army too, the partner is lying near me lethargic purple and blue. All the monsters locked into his intricate mind. If I wasn't prepared to believe in his fantasies, he will never make me his wife, he lies dying, his body crumbling away, fragile and broken, but *'Hiss will'* is fighting to stay:

"I will always love you! I will never let you go"

he whispers.

"If you will not marry me then no one will marry you!"

He metamorphosizes into the reptile and amphibian creatures changing shapes simultaneously in front of my eyes.

Hissing, spitting, growling, my partner shows all his monster forms as his body evolves and fades, with bluish black patches materialising through his flesh, and a devouring eating bug with razor slicing teeth is stripping his skin and muscles the raw bones protruding. The Hiss returns to squeeze my life away, the wolf howls the Komodo dragon spits his poison so hard in my face and throat I deathly banshee scream pain. The poison burns, my body collapses in a melted heap shrivelling away as I mutate into my manic monster changing partners decaying flesh. *He was my twin hell flame.* My mouth twisted open wide regurgitating stench mustard vomit over the dying partner who twisted my mind.

He wanted monster reptiles to rule the world,
but they chose to rule me as well.
The zombie nursing staff lurched forward stabbing both of us with syringes and knifes with venom, and then turning on each other, gouging hostile wars,
a fight to death because we breathed our vile head thoughts into them.

With my last dying breathe I thundered a bellowing deafening tone of defiance!

"FUCK YOU ALL! MONSTERS IN MY HEAD! THE PHOENIX WITHIN ME WILL RISE AGAIN!"

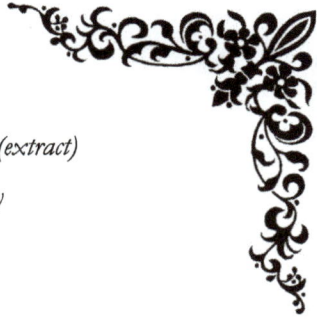

Positve Affirmations *(extract)*

By *Anne-Louise Lowrey*

Not ferocious not cruel
but brave and kind
the one who struggles with their mind.
Positive living good relations
I am wary of self-adoration
yet every day we get lovelier
and lovelier. All of us.
Write it on the mirror
the wardrobe door and in the porch
before you go out
don't leave yourself in doubt.
Happiness may sometimes
seem contrived little rays of joy
make the most of being alive.
When things are hard to bear
you look around there's no one there
but some-one can be found inside
the time is now come out of your hide.

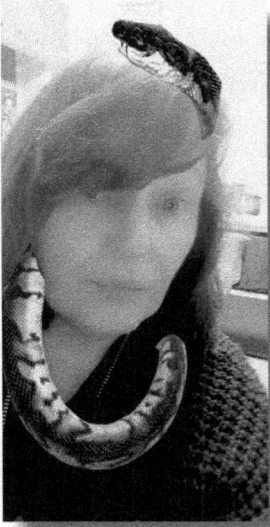

There is a moment in time to reflect on living and the losses it causes.
Writing is a release which empowers the soul to be stronger.

This story holds a memory of the past that was meant to be, and a future that can change the present by those who read THE HISS.

Alma Blair

www.ingramcontent.com/pod-product-compliance
Lightning Source LLC
Chambersburg PA
CBHW071632040426
42452CB00009B/1588